Caring for Family Members and Patients Who Need Us Because We Care

Information About Caring for Those with Alzheimer's Disease and Traumatic Brain Injury, Plus Dealing with Eldercare Abuse

FRAN LEWIS

This is an original pamphlet and guide for caregivers, volunteers and nurses and aides to use as resource when working with patients with Alzheimer's, dementia or any illness that involves memory loss. The author is not a doctor nor is she dispensing any medical advice. This guide has been created to help those who are caregivers or are thinking of volunteering in a hospital or nursing home facility.

You may reproduce this guide, with permission, to use for meetings and to train volunteers. You may not sell or use this for commercial benefit or profit.

Please contact the author at riffyone@optonline.net for permission to copy this document.

What people are saying about this book:

Fran Lewis has dealt with this difficult and complex issue with sensitivity both for the person with the condition and the caregiver. She has a deep understanding of the conditions involved, what the caregivers are facing, and how they can cope. I would highly recommend this book for everyone, not just those currently dealing with this situation. Unfortunately, others of us may face it in the future.

~ Allan Topol, award winning author of the Craig Page serious

This is a worthwhile read for anyone who finds themselves in caregiver mode. Giving a voice to millions of caregivers of patients with Alzheimer's Disease and traumatic brain injuries, this new work by Fran Lewis is heartfelt and touching. Lewis shares a glimpse of what caregivers endure during this illness—from tender compassion for their loved ones to the personal struggle of trying to help non-caregivers understand the depth of the illness. Lewis offers real-world tips from a patien tcare point of view, and she provides gentle reminders to help caregivers preserve some compassion for themselves.

~ Laura Wharton
Award-winning author of mysteries and a caregiver for her beloved
father, www.LauraWhartonBooks.com

I thought about a road trip when reading what you sent me. Dealing with your mother's disease and how you had no help with her. You gave some great tips on caregiving, and also some personal anecdotes.

~William Butler

Fran Lewis's book is truly amazing. She's been a caregiver throughout all the information and experiences she's gone through and explains it all to you. You are truly not alone when these challenges hit your family. Fran is so generous and loving with all of the thorough information she shares with you because she's been through it all. You now have a step by step empowering guide if and when your family is struck by this challenge. I volunteered with Alzheimer's and dementia patients, and I had my intuition to work with. Would have loved this book then. The same goes for families dealing with someone having a brain injury. I highly recommend you buy this book now.

~Sherri Rosen, Publicist, NYC

What happens when you suddenly become a caregiver for a loved one? Fran Lewis, the author of *Caring for Family Members and Patients Who Need Us: Because We Care* has written a guide filled with information about almost every contingency while you are a caregiver. She has also included the stories of several other people relating their own experiences. Fran is, unfortunately, an expert in this field, having been a caregiver dealing with her now deceased mother with Alzheimer's disease. She has written an entire book about this experience: *Memories Are Precious: Alzheimer's Journey: Ruth's Story*, which describes her mother's experiences and how, as her caregiver, she learned how to take care of her and herself in the process. In this new book, *Caring for Family Members and Patients Who Need Us*, Ms. Lewis includes ways for caregivers to help themselves and answers questions that rarely get answered for caregivers. She delves into the practices of nursing homes as well and gives ways to deal with them. This is the book to give anyone who is a caregiver.

~ Barbara Ehrentreu, Author of: *If I Could Be Like Jennifer Taylor, After and You'll Probably Forget Me Living With and Without Hal* and award winning screenwriter for "The Kiss"

Contents

PART TWO
Traumatic Brain Injury

PART ONE

Caregivers:
Why You Are So Special

Caregivers:
What You Need To Know

By Fran Lewis

In August of 2003 my family's life drastically changed. On August 25 of that year, my mom got sick. She woke up with a sharp pain in her back and could hardly breathe. She called my aunt and told her to come down to her apartment, and not to call my sister or me. She wanted to handle this without worrying either one of us. However, this was not to be.

My aunt called 911 and they responded to the call, but insisted that one of her children be present when they did the initial exam and assessment. I was and still am the only one who knows what meds my mom takes and how often, and the dosage.

After dealing with the preliminary issues and arriving at the hospital, the staff immediately addressed my mother's issues and concerns. They did numerous tests to find out what had caused her problem. From what she was saying, it sounded like she did not remember taking her blood thinner medicine and had overdosed on it by accident. She had always been very careful with her Coumadin. However, she had been forgetting to take it and was forgetting a lot more too. Frightening as this might seem, it only got worse.

From this hospital, she was taken by ambulance to another one, where they thought they could address what they believed was an aortic aneurysm. However, this was incorrect.

The following morning I received a call from the heart surgeon in charge of my mom's case, asking permission to operate before it was too late. Of course I did not hesitate, and allowed him to save her life. Fortunately, I got there just in time to see her before surgery. This was the last time she would sound lucid or clear for a very long time.

She came out of the operation with many more problems. She had died twice on the table and had to be revived. (I was told this later on.) She began to slur her words and not understand what was happening around her. The physical operation was a success, but her mental capacity for dealing with things and understanding what was happening around her were greatly diminished.

When she finally came home from the hospital two weeks later she had to reenter the next day due to complications that no one realized when she was discharged. Because of four more stays in the hospital, my family and I noticed that her ability to process information and deal with daily situations had been compromised by the surgery and the anesthesia that was given. She even realized that she could not remain alone for any long period.

Due to all of the stays in the hospital and many other factors that changed her ability to care for herself, we were forced to find help for her by enlisting VNS (Visiting Nurse Services) to find us aides to care for her the right way. Unfortunately, this turned out to be costly to my family and me. I had to change my lifestyle and my way of living, which no one seemed to care about. I had to retire from teaching early and find other interests that I could pursue at home. One, of course, was writing books, and the other short stories. I have even tried to publicize the fact that I am writing a book about Alzheimer's as a resource for other families to be able to learn more about this illness and to get the help and care they need for a loved one.

The only problem is that no one realizes that, as the person who has to deal with nurses, doctors, home care agencies, and home care providers, you still need to take time for yourself and have some kind of life. I have been nowhere for the last seven years since my mom was diagnosed with this awful illness.

She is getting much worse, and now rather than make her presence known she just sits and stares all day while sitting on her chair in front of her television. Although the aides do try, and sometimes succeed in taking her out in her wheelchair to get some air and possibly run into an old friend who might stop and say hello, she often rebels and refuses to leave her chair. It seems like it is her safety net, and she is afraid of anything that is different or change in general.

It is really hard to remain calm and neutral when it comes to other family members that go away on vacation and do not check and see how my mom is, or if there is something that I might have planned or need to do. They usually plan their flights or trips, and tell me about them when they have their trips finalized. This gets me quite upset and I often get into it with the other person. I try to explain that there are times that I would like to do something during the day, or even stay over in a hotel with my husband for the night. The home health aides are not allowed to give my mom her meds. I have to give them to her twice a day. I can put them together once in a while in the morning, but the pill she takes to stay calm should not be given in a double dose in the morning. She will be too calm and possibly sleep throughout the day, making it hard for the day aide to feed her.

People forget that caregivers might actually do other things during the day. So, when I state that I am busy writing an article for a magazine, or just for one of my books, or to post on one of the many sites that I belong to, people often say, "What are you busy with? You don't work." I work from home, and probably get more done in a day than they do working in an office. I never put anyone down and I respect whatever others do. I worked for over 36 years in the NYC Public Schools, and I miss working with the students in reading and writing everyday. I had fun teaching my writing classes, and working with students in reading and teaching the classics was not only fun, but also rewarding.

Caregivers are people too, and not just people who provide time and care for a person that is ill. Others need to understand that the caregiver needs time to regroup and regenerate him or herself and take time to feel

Caregivers Are Special People
Tips to Help You Survive

As the primary and only caregiver for my mom who has Alzheimer's, I have had to develop different ways to keep myself active and my mind stimulated. All too often as a caregiver we become so immersed in taking care of the needs of the person who is ill that we forget about our own. When you make the decision to care for the family member at home, you are really taking on a challenge of Herculean proportion. Everyday is different and every challenge unique, and must be handled differently but with kindness and care.

When a person has Alzheimer's the hardest thing to deal with is their forever changing erratic behaviors. They can be calm one minute and out of control or violent the next. These behaviors tend to put a lot of stress and strain on the caregiver. Here are some ways that I found work with my mom and might help others deal with these behaviors.

Discussions and tips

- I find that speaking slowly and softly in a calm voice does help to calm the person down.

- Speaking in simple sentences and short phrases does help.

- Repeating something in different ways sometimes helps her to understand what she needs to do. It is a simple as saying, "Open" or "Open your mouth" instead of, "Eat this" or trying to explain to her that she needs to eat.

- I always call her by her first name, or of course Mom, to get her attention: at this point she still knows who she is when you call her. She does not always say her name or respond verbally when asked who she is.

- Always be positive and smile at the person. Do not let them think that you are angry with them. They are not at fault, and cannot control or help their behaviors.

Cleaning and dressing the person

1. The one thing that is hard when trying to keep a person with this illness clean is trying to bathe the person. Fortunately, I do have four home health aides that are great. But, they often ask me to assist them when she is hard to handle. They told me they have daily schedule for bathing, feeding, and getting her dressed.

2. Always be kind and gentle when bathing the person, and always pick out clothing that is easy to put on and easy to get off.

3. Explain what you are going to do and why, even if the person does not fully understand.

4. They always make sure that they have the soap, sponges, and the showerhead ready when bathing her. She sits on a bench in the tub, which makes it safer and prevents her from falling. She has a railing up on the side so she cannot get out by herself.

5. If a shower is not possible using a handheld shower-head, then a sponge bath might be the next best option.

6. Dressing the person is often more difficult. You need to get the person dressed at the same time each day. It is important that the person, whether they are going out or not, should get dressed everyday. They need to have their hair and nails groomed and cleaned and look as normal as possible.

7. If the person with AD is still able to choose what they want to wear, then let them have the choice. It will make them feel better and show that they are being treated with respect and dignity.

8. I find that elastic waists in pants are easier for the aides to dress her.

9. Slip on shoes are the easier than tying knots in sneakers or walking shoes.

Eating

This can be a real challenge, especially in the late stages of the illness. Here are some tips to making that easier for you as the caregiver.

1. If the person is having trouble chewing certain foods or if the foods are hard to swallow, you can puree the foods in a blender, turning it into a softer consistency to be eaten. I find that when the aides make chicken soup and add pasta, potatoes, and other vegetables, it is easier for my mom to eat the soup if it is pureed.

2. If the person is aware of what they might want to eat you might give that person some choices. I would limit the choices to two, so as not to overwhelm the person with too much decision-making.

3. You need to choose foods that allow the person to eat independently, and hopefully without having to be fed or needing too much assistance.

4. The one thing that is vital is that since the amount of foods or food the person consumes will eventually

decrease as the disease progresses, you need to make sure that they drink a lot of fluids to prevent dehydration.

5. It is necessary to make sure that there is nothing in the foods that is difficult to swallow, because as the disease progresses it will become harder for the person to swallow and you need to prevent them from choking.

Incontinence

You need to make sure that the nurse assigned to the person who requires care knows which home care agency will provide the supplies needed on a monthly basis rather than having you pay for them out of pocket. You need to follow these tips, too.

1. Set up a daily schedule for the person to go to the bathroom. The aides change my mom every two hours to prevent rashes, sores, and chafing. They make sure that they have A&D ointment on hand, as well as Destin or BalmX, in order to make sure that she does not get any sores of any kind.

2. If the person starts to fidget and gets restless, that can often be sign that the person should be taken to the bathroom on the spot. (If they are still capable of using the bathroom.)

3. Be aware that accidents will happen, and you need to stay calm and be understanding. The first time this happened to my mom she was in the hospital and did realize that she was forgetting to go to the bathroom. She often rang for the nurse, who never came.

    I think part of her problem came because she just didn't get there in time, as well as the poor staffing on her floor of people that did not really concern themselves with patients that were incontinent. I know that they get busy and back up, but it became apparent that this was going to be an issue. She did not want to wear the diapers, and wanted to use the bedpan or the commode.

4. To prevent nighttime accidents, limit the amount of fluids the person drinks before going to bed.

5. If the person is aware of whether they need to use the bathroom and you are going on a long trip, you might want to learn where the rest stops are located on your route so you can stop. Have the person take extra clothes in case of an accident. I know that with my mom we made sure that she had a Depend or pull up diaper on top of her underwear to prevent this issue from causing her any embarrassment.

Sleeping and Wandering

1. My mom does not sleep through the night. When we first found out she had the illness she even tried to leave the apartment and go shopping in the middle of the night. She left one morning and walked to the bakery to get bread. Not really knowing where and why she did that, she stopped a stranger in a car to drive her home. Lucky for her the person knew her. When I got the call from the aide, who was late in coming to care for her, that she was missing and finally found, I realized that we needed more help and more hours too.

2. Make sure that you enroll the person in the Safe Return Program from the Alzheimer's Association. This is a program that helps you register the person with the necessary information needed to contact you in case the person gets lost. You receive two bracelets and a necklace, plus labels. You can sew the labels into the clothing of the person, and you can wear one bracelet and the person requiring care the other. In case of an emergency both parties can be helped and contacted.

3. Keep a photo of the person in your wallet, on a table in your living room, and in their home in case the person is lost and ID needs to be made by the police.

4. Keep a list of the person's medications and other vital information handy, including how much medication is prescribed and how often the pills are taken. Post on the refrigerator or another conspicuous place, along with their plan of care if you have home care.

5. Make sure that you put sharp objects out of their reach. Unplug toaster ovens and microwaves because they might forget to turn them off when they try to use them. Prepare meals for them and leave them in the refrigerator to be warmed by you or an aide. Make sure that the locks on the front door are too high for the person to open. Make sure if there is a back door that it is secured and locked and cannot be opened. You might want to have a keyed deadbolt or an additional lock, which is too high for the person to reach, placed on the front door of a house or an apartment. You might even add a chain.

6. These people get disoriented and cannot tell the difference between day and night. Assure them that they are in a safe place and safe environment. Never yell at them, scold them, or make them feel like they did something wrong. Remember: It is the disease, NOT THEM causing these behaviors.

7. As the disease gets worse the person might begin seeing things, hearing things, and have delusions. Hallucinations are when the person sees, hears, smells, and feels that something or someone is there but it really is not.

8. Delusions are beliefs that are false from which the person is so totally convinced that something is happening they cannot be dissuaded.

Never yell at the person, and assure them that you are taking care of getting rid of whatever is upsetting them. I remember my Aunt Tova was given Haldol in the hospital and thought she saw squirrels on the ceiling of her room and that she had left old bread and cheese in her freezer. She made my cousin call me, and I told her that I would get rid of the bread and cheese and was right there to take care of the squirrels. She even told me she saw my Uncle Irving and my father Doc, who had been gone a long time.

You Count Too!

Remember to make time for yourself and your family. Do not neglect your personal appearance or your personal needs. Make sure that you take time for yourself every day. Make sure that you develop an interest or a hobby and set aside time, as I do, to pursue what makes you happy.

Make sure that when you feel stressed you take a break and go out for a walk, rest, or just read a book. You cannot be on 24 hours a day. Make sure that if the person needs an aide that you get the services needed in order to help you have some kind of life and time with your family.

I know that there is always one person in a family that gets the burden of the care. That, of course, is not right and not fair. However, you need to make sure that you get to go away even overnight or on a weekend in order to rejuvenate yourself and feel better. You deserve it. I know I need time off from giving my mom her meds every morning and every night. I sometimes feel like I am wearing a straight jacket that needs to be loosened. I wish that I could go away for a week, but I know that is not in the cards. No one wants the responsibility of dealing with the agencies and the meds and the aides. It gets tough.

But, as I have been told so many times, I am doing the right thing, and someday I will be blessed and rewarded. I can look myself in the mirror and know that I have nothing to be guilty about, and know that I am trying my best to keep my mom at home. I know that a person with AD has a limited life style. I promised her that I would never put her in a facility of any kind, and I will not break that promise.

How Do You Know When You Need to Get Help for a Loved One?

When my mom went shopping by herself to the bakery one morning and asked a total stranger to drive her home, I knew things were taking a downward slide. Asking her why she would accept a ride with someone she did not know, she looked at me and said, "I have no idea what you are talking about. That lady is my friend." She was a friend whose name she did not know, nor did I.

When my mom began to exhibit the following behaviors, my brother, sister, and I realized we needed to get her more help than the three of us could provide. This is where you need to do research and a lot of legwork to make sure that you get the right help for your parent or loved one.

1. When someone is unable to remember things

2. Asking or repeating the same question or story multiple times

3. Lost in familiar places

4. Being unable to follow and understand directions

5. Getting disoriented about time, people, and places

6. Neglecting personal safety, hygiene, and nutrition

7. As in my mom's case, asking a stranger for a ride home

8. Wandering the neighborhood and not remembering their own address

9. Forgetting names and places

10. As in my mom's case, taking her meds more than the required number of times a day

Kindness tips

1. Always say good morning when entering a patient's room.

2. Address the patient by name and tell the patient your name.

3. SMILE!

4. Explain the task you are going to perform before you do it, and explain the task as you are performing. Patients are often leery or afraid of strangers, and need to feel confident and safe with you.

5. If a patient needs assistance bathing, eating, or walking, help them and do not leave them before they complete the task.

6. Patients that need help eating: You need to make sure that person eats and is fed. Make sure that you do not leave the tray untouched, and if you have to feed the patient you need to do it with kindness and patience.

7. Ask the patient if they need help dressing, or assistance going to breakfast or any other area of the home or hospital.

8. If you are bringing magazines or books, allow the person to choose.

9. Never speak to a patient as if they were a small child.

10. Speak to people with respect and as an adult.

11. Make sure that the person's environment is safe.

12. Make sure you have a list of things that need to be done for that person and complete them.

13. Meet with other volunteers and discuss their successes.

14. When you speak to a patient, make sure that you make eye contact and have their attention.

15. Speak at eye level and speak clearly.

16. Use simple and direct statements.

17. Never raise your voice.

18. Include the person in your conversation: Talk to the person, not at the person.

19. Never speak to them as if they are a third party and not in the same room.

20. Listen to their concerns and show a lot of understanding.

21. Never leave a patient in distress.

Your role is important and valuable

There are many jobs that are special and important. Never think that because you are not getting paid as a volunteer that it hinders your value, importance, or role. Many of the people you come in contact with have no family members visiting, are afraid to be alone, and might look forward to your visit, no matter how long or short, as the highlight of their day. Just walking into their room and knowing that you are there to speak to them, perform a needed task, or just sit and talk with them can be the difference between someone giving up on life and feeling needed and special.

Everything you do has value and a purpose. Never allow anyone to tell you that you do not have be work or volunteer on a specific day, because it does not matter since you are not getting paid. Work ethics need to be adhered to. Volunteer positions can lead to paying ones. You never know. Your time is valuable, and what you are doing to help someone that is in these facilities is worth more than all the money in the world. Never sell what you are doing short.

Remember:

- Remember to be sensitive to the needs of the person.

- Understand that the diagnosis is upsetting and show compassion.

- Remember to speak to the person as an adult and a human being, and not a small child.

- Communicate with the Alzheimer's patient.

- Have an upbeat and positive attitude.

- Understand and learn how to handle behavior changes.

- Expect that the patient will have memory loss, and over time even more.

- Get support for yourself and make sure that you do not neglect you.

- Speak in short, familiar words, phrases, and simple sentences. Repeat yourself if necessary. Stay calm.

- Allow the person plenty of time to answer. If the person does not respond or answer, reword the question.

- Ask only one question at a time.

- Never give negative instructions. Do not say "Don't" or "Never" or "You'd better not." Say "Let's try this" or "Let's go over here."

- We are in this together!

- Work together and help them understand.

- Mobility is important, and your assistance makes a big difference.

- Shopping can help them stay focused and feeling useful.

- Your visit and care makes all the difference.

- Helping someone with a smile makes a difference in the other person's life.

Remember: Everything you do matters and is special. Caregivers are special and unique!

Resources that I used for this pamphlet:

www.alz.org

www.nia.nih.gov

www.nia.nih.gov/Alzheimers

www.nia.nih.gov/Alzheimers/Publications/caregiverguide.htm#intro

www.nia.nih.gov/Healthinformation/Publications/forgetfulness.htm

Important information

1. What are the signs of memory loss?

2. What are the stages of the disease?

3. What can you do when you are diagnosed with it?

4. What are the changes in behaviors?

5. What safety measures can you take at home?

6. What personal care changes occur and need to be addressed?

7. Caregiver Information

8. Supporting the caregiver

9. Resources to get help and support

10. Changes in eating and sleeping

Ten warning signs of Alzheimer's disease*

The Alzheimer's Association has developed the following list of warning signs that include common symptoms of Alzheimer's disease. Individuals who exhibit several of these symptoms would see a physician for a complete evaluation.

1. Memory loss

2. Difficulty performing familiar tasks

3. Problems with language

4. Disorientation to time and place

5. Poor or decreased judgment

6. Problems with abstract thinking

7. Misplacing things

8. Changes in mood or behavior

9. Changes in personality

10. Loss of initiative

*This information comes from www.medicine.net.com

It is normal for certain kinds of memory, such as the ability to remember lists of words, to decline with normal aging. In fact, normal individuals fifty years of age will recall only about 60% as many times on some kinds of memory tests as individuals twenty years of age. Every 20 year old is well aware of multiple times he or she could not think of an answer on a test that he or she once knew. But, most 20 year olds do not worry about forgetting something or that he or she has the early stages of Alzheimer's. But, a person 50 or 60 years of age with a few memory lapses may worry that they have the early stages of the disease.

This information came from the Alzheimer's Association Pamphlet: Basics of Alzheimer's disease: what it is and what can you do.

Many of us notice slowed or delayed thinking or that we have difficulty remembering things. However, serious memory loss, confusion, and other major changes in the way our minds work are not a normal part of aging.

There are many conditions that disrupt memory and mental function. These symptoms may improve when the underlying cause is treated.

Possible reasons or causes for memory loss:

1. Depression
2. Medication side effects
3. Excess use of alcohol
4. Thyroid problems
5. Poor diet
6. Vitamin deficiencies
7. Certain infections
8. Alzheimer's disease and related dementias

What is the difference between someone with Alzheimer's and someone with normal age related memory changes?

If you experience significant memory problems you need to see a doctor. Early diagnosis and intervention methods are improving, and treatment options and sources of support can improve your quality of life.

Someone with Alzheimer's

- Forgets whole experiences

- Rarely remembers later

- Is gradually unable to follow written/spoken directions

- Is gradually unable to use notes

- Is gradually unable to care for self

Someone with normal age-related memory changes

- Forgets part of an experience

- Often remembers later

- Is usually able to follow written/spoken directions

- Is usually able to use notes

- Is usually able to care for self

These are 10 signs of Alzheimer's disease

1. **Memory loss:** You forget recently learned information: this is a mot common early sign of dementia. You begin to forget more often and are unable to recall information later.

2. **Difficulty performing familiar tasks:** People with dementia often find it hard to plan or finish everyday tasks. These people may lose track of the steps involved in preparing a meal, placing a phone call, or playing a game.

3. **Problems with Language:** People with Alzheimer's disease often forget simple words or substitute unusual

words, making their speech or writing hard to understand. They may be unable to find the toothbrush, and may ask for that thing for my mouth instead.

4. **Disorientation to time and place:** People with this disease can become lost in their own neighborhoods, forget where they are and how they got there, and not know how to get back home.

5. **Poor or decreased judgment:** People with the disease often dress inappropriately, wearing many layers on a warm day and or little clothing in the cold. They may show poor judgment about money by giving away large amount to telemarketers over the phone.

6. **Problems with abstract thinking:** Some with Alzheimer's disease may have unusual trouble performing complex mental tasks, like forgetting what numbers are and how they should be used.

7. **Misplacing things:** A person with this disease may put things in unusual places. This person might put an iron in the freezer or a wristwatch in the refrigerator.

8. **Changes in mood or behavior:** Someone with this disease may show rapid mood swings—from calm to tears to anger—for no apparent reason.

9. **Changes in Personality:** The personalities of people with dementia can change dramatically. They may become extremely confused, suspicious, fearful or dependent on a family member.

10. **Loss of initiative:** A person with this disease may become very passive, sitting in front of the TV for hours, sleeping more than usual, or not wanting to do usual activities.

What is normal?

1. Forgetting names or appointments occasionally

2. Occasionally forgetting why you came into a room or what you planned to do

3. Sometimes having trouble finding the right word

4. Forgetting the day of the week or where you were going

5. Making questionable or debatable decisions from time to time

6. Challenging to balance a checkbook

7. Misplacing keys or a wallet temporarily

8. Occasionally feeling sad or moody

9. People's personalities do change somewhat with age

10. Sometimes feeling weary of work or social obligations.

Doctor Discussion Guide

Your family member may be concerned about the changes mentioned in the previous section that might indicate mild to moderate Alzheimer's disease of dementia.

The following information comes from the website of Novartis. These are the questions that you need to ask your doctor.

1. Do the symptoms indicate a problem?

2. Is Alzheimer's disease dementia one of the possible things that might be causing these symptoms?

3. Are there other conditions that might be causing these symptoms?

4. Will tests be needed in order for you to make this diagnosis? Which ones?

5. How long will it be before I will know the diagnosis?

6. If it is Alzheimer's disease, what should I expect?

7. What medicines are available?

8. Can these medicines help slow the worsening of symptoms? Which ones?

9. How do these medicines work?

These are questions your doctor might ask you or a family member*:

1. Are you or someone you care for:

   a. Forgetting conversations, appointments, or holidays?

   b. Having difficulty finding the right words to express their thoughts or your thoughts?

   c. Repeating stories or questions?

   d. Getting lost in familiar places?

2. Have you or someone you care for:

   a. Forgotten how to do familiar activities, like cooking or repairing things?

   b. Had difficulty doing bills or balancing the checkbook, or thrown away a bill before paying it?

   c. Been misplacing things more often than usual?

3. Have you or someone you care for:

   a. Lost interest in friends, hobbies, or other activities that were once enjoyable?

   b. Been resisting change or new activities?

   c. Become more upset or angrier than usual?

   d. Often felt sad?

*This information comes from the Alzheimer's Association

People with memory loss or other possible warning signs of Alzheimer's may fail to recognize that they have a problem and might resist following up on their symptoms. Signs of dementia may be more obvious to friends and family.

The first step is to find a doctor you feel comfortable with. Your local Alzheimer's Association can assist you with finding a doctor. There is no one type of doctor that specializes in diagnosing and treating this disease. Many people usually contact their primary care doctor about their concerns. Primary care doctors often oversee the diagnostic process themselves.

Another problem people face when diagnosed with this disease is how the doctor or medical profession explains the illness and how the person is told. It heartbreaking enough for anyone to be told that this is happening to them and that their future is no longer in their control. The Alzheimer's Association suggested this to ease the way for the person and family to understand what is going to happen, and to give the person a dignified diagnosis.

1. **Speak to the patient directly**—that is the person with dementia. They are the person with the disease, and the person that needs to know and understand first.

2. **Tell the truth.** Doctors do not always have all of the answers, but they should be honest about what they do know and why they believe the knowledge they have is the truth.

3. **Test early.** The patient needs an accurate diagnosis as fast as possible, which gives them more time to deal and live to their fullest potential. It gives the person time to get more information about the appropriate clinical trials.

4. **Take the patient's concerns seriously, regardless of their age.** Age may be the biggest risk factor for this disease. It is definitely not a normal part of aging. Do not make the patient feel that their concerns are unfounded, or they are old so they do not understand what is happening to them. This disease can hit people in their 40s, 50s, and 60s.

5. **Deliver the news in plain but sensitive language.** This is probably one of the most vital and important things that the patient needs to hear. Using language that the person can understand and is sensitive will help the person feel better, and know that the health care provider is showing compassion for his/her feelings

6. **Coordinate with other care providers.** If the patient is seeing more than one specialist, it is important that the doctors coordinate their information so that any changes in the patient can be identified early on, and that they do not have to retake or repeat any tests unnecessarily.

7. **Explain the purpose of different tests and what you hope to learn from them.** These tests can be both physically and emotionally draining. It helps the patient to understand the purpose of all of the tests and the duration of each test, and what you hope to learn from them. There should be an option for the patient to take a breather or a break between tests that are longer in order to ask questions.

8. **Do not give the patient this diagnosis and leave them alone to deal with it.** The person needs to understand what is going to happen to them, and they need to know if there are any medical options and what support services are available for them and their family members.

9. **Work with the patient on a plan for healthy living.**

10. **Give recommendations for keeping healthy.** Medication may help modify some of the neurological symptoms. Other recommendations for keeping healthy include diet, exercise, and social engagements.

11. **Recognize that the patient is an individual and will experience the disease in his/her own unique way.** This disease affects each person in different ways and at a different rate. Telling the patient the rate that this illness will affect him/her and how fast things will go

downhill needs to be addressed to that patient, and not to others in general.

12. **Alzheimer's is a journey, not a destination.** There is no prescription to cure this illness, and doctors need to be their patient's advocate and work with them to get quality care and try to have some type of life while going through these changes.

Stages of Alzheimer's disease

Experts have documented common patterns of symptom progression that occur in many individuals with Alzheimer's disease, and developed several methods of "staging" based on these patterns. Progression of symptoms corresponds in a general way to the underlying nerve cell degeneration that takes place in Alzheimer's disease.

Nerve cell damage typically begins with cells involved in learning and memory, and gradually spreads to cells that control other aspects of thinking, judgment, and behavior. The damage eventually affects cells that control and coordinate movement.

Staging systems provides useful frames of reference for understanding how the disease may unfold and for making future plans. But it is important to note that all stages are artificial benchmarks in a continuous process that can vary greatly from one person to another. Not everyone will experience every symptom, and symptoms may occur at different times in different individuals. People with Alzheimer's die an average of four to six years after diagnosis, but the duration of the disease can vary from three to 20 years.

The framework for this fact sheet is a system that outlines key symptoms characterizing seven stages, ranging from unimpaired function to very severe cognitive decline. This framework is based on a system developed by Barry Reisberg, M.D., Clinical Director of the New York University School of Medicine's Silberstein Aging and Dementia Research Center.

Within this framework, we have noted which stages correspond to the widely used concepts of mild, moderate, moderately severe, and severe Alzheimer's disease. We have also noted which stages fall within the more general divisions of early-stage, mid-stage, and late-stage categories.

Stage 1: No cognitive impairment

Unimpaired individuals experience no memory problems, and none are evident to a health care professional during a medical interview.

Stage 2: Very mild decline

Individuals at this stage feel as if they have memory lapses, forgetting familiar words or names or the location of keys, eyeglasses, or other everyday objects. But these problems are not evident during a medical examination or apparent to friends, family, or co-workers.

Stage 3: Mild cognitive decline

Early-stage Alzheimer's can be diagnosed in some, but not all, individuals with these symptoms. Friends, family, or co-workers begin to notice deficiencies. Problems with memory or concentration may be measurable in clinical testing or discernible during a detailed medical interview. Common difficulties include:

- Word or name-finding problems noticeable to family or close associates
- Decreased ability to remember names when introduced to new people
- Performance issues in social and work settings noticeable to others
- Reading a passage and retaining little material
- Losing or misplacing a valuable object
- Decline in ability to plan or organize

Stage 4: Moderate cognitive decline
(Mild or early-stage Alzheimer's disease)

At this stage, a careful medical interview detects clear-cut deficiencies in the following areas:

- Decreased knowledge of recent events
- Impaired ability to perform challenging mental arithmetic. For example, to count backward from 100 by 7s

- Decreased capacity to perform complex tasks, such as marketing, planning dinner for guests, or paying bills and managing finances
- Reduced memory of personal history
- The affected individual may seem subdued and withdrawn, especially in socially or mentally challenging situations

Stage 5: Moderately severe cognitive decline
(Moderate or mid-stage Alzheimer's disease)

Major gaps in memory and deficits in cognitive function emerge. Some assistance with day-to-day activities becomes essential. At this stage, individuals may:

- Be unable during a medical interview to recall such important details as their current address, their telephone number, or the name of the college or high school from which they graduated
- Become confused about where they are or about the date, day of the week, or season
- Have trouble with less challenging mental arithmetic; for example, counting backward from 40 by 4s or from 20 by 2s
- Need help choosing proper clothing for the season or the occasion

- Usually retain substantial knowledge about themselves and know their own name and the names of their spouse or children

- Usually require no assistance with eating or using the toilet

Stage 6: Severe cognitive decline
(Moderately severe or mid-stage Alzheimer's disease)

Memory difficulties continue to worsen, significant personality changes may emerge, and affected individuals need extensive help with daily activities. At this stage, individuals may:

- Lose most awareness of recent experiences and events, as well as of their surroundings

- Recollect their personal history imperfectly, although they generally recall their own name

- Occasionally forgets the name of their spouse or primary caregiver, but generally can distinguish familiar from unfamiliar faces

- Need help getting dressed properly; without supervision, may make such errors as putting pajamas over daytime clothes or shoes on wrong feet; experience disruption of their normal sleep/waking cycle

- Need help with handling details of toileting (flushing toilet, wiping, and disposing of tissue properly)

- Have increasing episodes of urinary or fecal incontinence

- Experience significant personality changes and behavioral symptoms, including suspiciousness and delusions (for example, believing that their caregiver is an impostor); hallucinations (seeing or hearing things that are not really there); or compulsive, repetitive behaviors such as hand wringing or tissue shredding

- Tend to wander and become lost

Stage 7: Very severe cognitive decline
(Severe or late-stage Alzheimer's disease)

This is the final stage of the disease, when individuals lose the ability to respond to their environment, the ability to speak, and, ultimately, the ability to control movement.

- Frequently individuals lose their capacity for recognizable speech, although words or phrases may occasionally be uttered

- Individuals need help with eating and toileting, and there is general incontinence

- Individuals lose the ability to walk without assistance, then the ability to sit without support, the ability to smile, and the ability to hold their head up. Reflexes become abnormal and muscles grow rigid. Swallowing is impaired.

Information for this section of the book was gleaned from information published by the Alzheimer's Association, 1.800.272.3900 | www.alz.org.

Groups and services

Here is information about support groups, services and information you might need to get the help and services you need.

1. Alzheimer's Disease Educations and Referral (ADEAR) Center, P.O. Box 8250, Silver Springs, MD, 20907-8250, 1-800-438-4380, www.alzheimers.nia.nih.gov

   This service of the National Institute of Aging offers information and publications on diagnosis, treatment, patient caregiver needs, long-term care, education and training; research related to AD. Staff answer telephone, e-mail, and written requests and make referrals to local and national resources.

2. Alzheimer's Association, 225 N. Michigan Avenue, Suite 1700, Chicago, IL 60601-7633, 1-800-272-3900, www.alz.org

   This nonprofit association supports families and caregivers of patients with Alzheimer's disease and funds research. Chapters nationwide provide referrals to local resources and services. They sponsor support groups and educational programs.

3. Children of Aging Parents, P.O. Box 167, Richboro, PA 18954, 1-800-227-7294, www.caps4caregivers.org

    This is a nonprofit group that provides information and materials for adults caring for their older parents. Caregivers of people with this disease might find their resources and information helpful.

4. Eldercare Locator, 1-800-677-1116, www.eldercare.gov

    This service of the Administration of Aging, funded by the Federal Government, provides information and referrals to respite care and other home and community services offered by State and Area Agencies on aging.

5. Family Caregiver Alliance, 180 Montgomery Street, Suite 1100, San Francisco, CA 94104, 1-800-445-8106, www.caregiver.org

    Family Caregiver Alliance is a community-based non-profit organization offering support services for those caring for adults and AD, stroke, traumatic brain injuries, and other cognitive disorders. Programs and services include an Information Clearinghouse fro FCA's publications.

Telling others about an Alzheimer's diagnosis

When you learn that someone you care about has Alzheimer's, you may hesitate to tell the person that he or she has the disease. You may also have a hard time deciding whether to tell family and friends. Once you are emotionally ready to discuss the diagnosis, how will you break the news? Here are some suggestions for talking about the disease with others.

Respect the person's right to know:

- You may want to protect the person by withholding information. But your loved one is an adult with the right to know the truth. It can be a relief to hear the diagnosis, especially if the person had suspected he or she had Alzheimer's disease.

- In many cases, people who are diagnosed early are able to participate in important decisions about their health-care and legal and financial planning.

- While there is no current cure for Alzheimer's, life will not stop with the diagnosis. There are treatments and services that can make life better for everyone.

Plan how to tell the person

- Talk with doctors, social workers, and others who work with people who have Alzheimer's to plan an approach for discussing the diagnosis.

- Consider a "family conference" to tell the person about the diagnosis. He or she may not remember the discussion, but may remember that people cared enough to come together. You may need to have more than one meeting to cover the details.

- Shape the discussion to fit the person's emotional state, medical condition, and ability to remember and make decisions.

- Pick the best time to talk about the diagnosis. People with Alzheimer's may be more receptive to new information at different times of the day.

- Don't provide too much information at once. Listen carefully to the person. They often signal the amount of information they can deal with through their questions and reactions. Later, you can explain the symptoms of Alzheimer's and talk about planning for the future and getting support. Help the person accept the diagnosis; the person may not understand the meaning of the diagnosis or may deny it. Accept such reactions and avoid further explanations. If they respond well, try providing additional information. The person with Alzheimer's may forget the initial discussion, but not the emotion involved. If telling them upsets them, hearing additional details may trigger the same reaction later.

- Reassure your loved one. Express your commitment to help and give support. Let the person know that you will do all you can to keep your lives fulfilling.

- Be open to the person's need to talk about the diagnosis and his or her emotions.

- Look for nonverbal signs of sadness, anger, or anxiety. Respond with love and reassurance.

- Encourage the person to join a support group for individuals with memory loss. Your local Alzheimer's Association can help you locate a group. To find an Association near you, please call 1.800.272.3900 or go to www.alz.org.

Telling family and friends

An Alzheimer diagnosis doesn't only affect the person receiving it. The lives of family members and friends may also drastically change.

- Be honest with family and friends about the person's diagnosis. Explain that Alzheimer's is a brain disease, not a psychological or emotional disorder.

- Share educational materials from the Alzheimer's Association. The more that people learn about the disease, the more comfortable they may feel around the person.

- Invite family to support groups sponsored by your local Alzheimer's Association.

- Realize that some people may drift out of your life, as they may feel uncomfortable around the person or may not want to help provide care.

- Alzheimer's disease can also impact children and teens. Just as with any family member, be honest about the person's diagnosis with the young people in your life.

- Encourage them to ask questions.

Information for this section of the book was gleaned from information published by the Alzheimer's Association, 1.800.272.3900 | www.alz.org.

Websites and information

- www.alz.org

- www.medicinenet.com/alzheimers_disease/page8.htm

- Fisher Center for Alzheimer's, www.alzinfo.org/alzheimers-treatment-overview.as;#3

- www.exelonpatch.com/info/For_the_Caregiver/saftey.jsp

Help to find the services you need:

1. Medicare

2. Visiting Nurse Service will come in and evaluate the patient for services to start and then help you to get Medicaid for your friend or family member.

3. Your local Congressman can help with some of their staff members who are trained to help you get the additional services you might need or to keep services that you already have in place.

Final Care

What You Need to Know
When the End is Near

The most difficult stage, of course, of any illness is the final one leading to the passing of the loved one. Whether Alzheimer's or any other terminal illness, twenty hour care seven days a week is apparent and needed. Caregivers need to realize that the last stage of Alzheimer's is difficult and very challenging. End of life decisions now have to be made, and final arrangements should be in place.

Understanding and anticipating what is to come is vital. Even with the most loving and outstanding care the end result is still the same. In this horrific last stage, the patient or loved one will lack the ability to communicate directly or verbally interact, will be totally dependent on the home health aides for all personal care, and will be confined to their bed or lift chair 24/7.

My mom no longer walks, although she has use of her limbs. She cannot stand or walk, even with a walker for balance. Most patients cannot recognize familiar pictures, people, or objects. However, if you show my mom some really old pictures from the past, at times she does remember the figures in them. Dependency on others becomes their way of life.

As in my mom's case, it is vital that she receives professional care from those trained and qualified to handle care for Alzheimer's patients. Although I monitor the care, administer her meds twice a day, and handle all of the paperwork required by Medicare and Medicaid, and the home health care agencies, without the four aides that so brilliantly and lovingly care for her I do not know what I would do, nor could I sleep at night. But, my cell phone is always on and right next to me if needed.

As a caregiver or even an aide, there are four important areas that must be stressed:

1. All practical care and assistance related to dressing, feeding, bathing, must be handled daily by the aides or caregiver. Skills-task and routines need to be carefully charted, listed, and recorded, either on a plan of care or by the caregiver, and taped on the refrigerator or other conspicuous place.

2. Speak to the patient politely, lovingly, and treat the person with respect and dignity in a nurturing environment so they feel safe and secure.

3. As a caregiver you are going to need help, support, or aid from other family members, health agents, legal and financial advisors.

4. Grief Support: after losing your loved one you might need counseling or to join a grief support group.

Other considerations:

1. Decide on whether you will keep the person at home or in a facility.

2. Seek financial and legal advice while the person can participate.

3. Hospice Services

4. Rabbi-priest-chaplain-clergy to speak with for support

5. Wills—living will

6. Family Conflicts: End of life directives need to be spelled out in writing, witnessed, and notarized by the patient before it is too late for them to make that vital decision.

7. Bereavement support

8. Implementing decisions for or against prolonged life treatments

Frequently Asked Questions:
Alzheimer's

1. Is it hereditary?

2. How can I find out if I am going to have it or have the gene?

3. What causes the plague to develop in the brain?

4. What about too much anesthesia?

5. Can diet and exercise delay or prevent the onset of the illness or the illness entirely?

6. Can it ever be reversed?

7. What research is being done and what are the latest medications that are being used or tested other than Namenda and Aricept?

8. What are the major warning signs?

9. How do I know what is normal and when I should be concerned?

10. When do I need help?

11. What agencies provide the answers?

12. Where Can I learn about support groups?

These questions and any that you have of your own need to be with you when you speak to your doctor or your family member's doctor?

Plus:

- Medications and how they are monitored

- When to stop the person from driving and take away the keys?

- When is 24 /7 care vital?

My mom drove me to the doctor one morning. Going home, she made a U-Turn down a one-way street and passed three red lights, and then turned down a one-way street to get home faster. When I tried to tell her she was going the wrong way, she told me she knew what she was doing. At that point, three police cars surrounded us. I thought I was living an episode of some cop show on television. I did not know whether to laugh or cry.

When the officers approached the car and told my mom what she had done, she answered them, "I did nothing wrong. What is your problem?"

Added to that, she was not wearing a seatbelt and proceeded to show them her scar from her heart surgery, saying the belt hurt her chest. When she looked for her license and car insurance, she could not find her current insurance even though it was in her wallet with her ten thousand other cards.

She then told me to flirt with the officers, even though I had a headache and was feeling crappy, to try and get them to not give her a ticket. By the time she got done, instead of eight tickets for eight violations, they let her off with a warning. It was at that point I called my sister and said it was time to take away Mom's keys. She parked the car, only to call my Aunt Tova to go to the supermarket later that day. She is a trip.

PART TWO

Traumatic Brain Injury

Protecting Your Brain

What You Need to Know and Understand About Traumatic Brain Injury and More

Traumatic Brain Injury

1. How to avoid brain injuries.

2. What safety precautions should you knows about and takes?

3. How are they treated?

4. What are the permanent effects?

5. What resources are out there to help if you have a traumatic brain injury?

An injury to your brain can result in loss of function and results in brain cell death. Traumatic brain injury is an external trauma to the head. It can also be caused by a violent movement of the head as a result of a fall, car crash, or being shaken.

When I was 17, I was in a serious car accident on a back road going to South Fallsburg. 'Til this day, I cannot tell you what really happened or who was at fault. All I remember is that I was sitting in the center seat in the rear of the car with my cousin and the driver's son. The driver and a friend of my mom were in the front two seats. My cousin and I sat quietly in the back of the car. We were going shopping for our mothers, and were really concentrating on the scenery and not talking about anything in particular.

As we rounded a corner on this back road another car was coming directly at us, and the next thing I remember, which was not a lot, was lights out. Someone yelled, "Look out!" but I guess not fast or loud enough.

It was a fatal head-on collision causing the person in the front passenger seat to die instantly, and I was thrown from the back of the car through the windshield and back.

The next thing I remember was sitting on a bench on a porch, having been pulled out of the wreck by an unknown person. Coming out of my stupor, I looked around and did not even recognize my surroundings or that I was severely injured.

My head hurt, my memory seemed fogged, and I had no idea who the people were sitting near me. My cousin tried to tell me who she was, and so did the son of the driver, but I just stared back at them, afraid. I kept asking more questions about what had happened, where we were going, and who they were, but nothing seemed to click.

What saved me from instant death was the fall (long flowing hair piece popular in the sixties and seventies) I was wearing on my head stuffed with sanitary napkins to add height, which must have cushioned the hard blow to my head. I later found out that I suffered a severe concussion, amnesia, blood clots, and hematomas on my legs and more. There were no SEAT BELTS in the back of the car, and the passenger and driver in the front were not buckled in.

My mother's friend died of a broken neck: she had no chance. The driver of the other car had leg injuries, my cousin lost her teeth, and the others had minor injuries.

Traumatic brain injury is serious and can have lasting results. But, car crashes are not the only causes of TBI. Bicycle accidents, sports injuries, severe falls, acts of violence, blows to the head, and even gunshot wounds are causes of TBI. The purpose of this article is to make you aware of the causes and how to prevent TBI.

Avoiding traumatic brain injury requires adhering to certain safety precautions when driving, engaging in sports activities, and even exercising. It is a simple as wearing a seat belt in a car whether in the passenger or driver's seat, or wearing a helmet when riding a bike. Here are some important tips or suggestions that might save your life.

Everyone needs to be safety conscious. These tips are not just for children, adults should heed them too. Your head is not a rubber ball and will not bounce back into place if injured. If you fall, get hit hard, or even worse, get shot, you might never recover. If you're racing cars, riding a bike, a horse, scooter, skateboard, snowboarding, or skiing, you need to wear a helmet. It's a simple as buckling up your seatbelt in a car, truck, or van. Sitting in your seat on a bus or a train. Using booster seats and properly fitted car seats for children.

Do not get behind the wheel of any vehicle if you are drunk or have taken any type of prescription drugs that make you tired. Never drive under the influence of any other kind of drug either.

Wear helmets when participating in sports: biking, riding a motorcycle, snowmobile, all-terrain vehicles, or even playing contact sports like football, soccer, boxing, and hockey should require wearing a helmet. When up at bat in a baseball game, wear that HELMET!

Horseback riding or being in a riding competition is fun, but you should wear a helmet in case of being thrown by the horse.

Skiing, snowboarding: Wear that helmet.

How to remain safe at home

1. Accidents can happen anywhere. Just because you are at home cooking in the kitchen or showering in the bath-

room does not mean that something might not happen. Walking on a torn or frayed carpet or area rug, or a wet mat that is not secured and doesn't have the proper rubber tips on it can cause a fall almost anywhere in your home.

2. Step stools should have grab bars on them to reach items that are high up in cabinets.

3. Windows should have window guards when small children live there, and they should be properly locked, as well as terrace or patio doors that are on high floors.

4. When vacuuming beware of the cord and make sure that your feet/legs do not become tangled as you move the machine about.

5. Install handrails on staircases.

6. Install safety gates at the top and bottom of stairs when young children are present. Keep gates locked.

7. Flames on stoves should not be left on without something cooking on them, and burners should not be left unattended.

8. Remove tripping hazards like small rugs. Mats are dangerous, and welcome mats can cause accidents too.

9. Use non-slip mats with tabs in the bathroom.

10. Grab bars should be installed in the shower or tub.

11. Exercise

12. Make sure your vision is checked.

13. If you have playground equipment in your backyard, make sure that every safety precaution is taken, and make sure you have the equipment regularly checked out.

14. The surface of the playground should be made of absorbing material like hardwood, mulch, or sand

15. Make sure that swings, slides, monkey bars, and other equipment is checked, and that chains that keep them sturdy are properly secured and the slides are not wobbly as children go down. Make sure the hand-rails are secured.

Symptoms of traumatic brain injury

Believe it or not, statistics have proved that every 21 seconds someone in the United States sustains traumatic brain injury. Americans suffer from head injuries on an annual basis, and over 80,000 of these are irreversible. According to the Centers for Disease Control and Prevention, head injuries are the leading cause of death in young adults and children. Forty percent of all injury related deaths in the United States are head injuries. After suffering a memory loss and severe head injury in a fatal car accident, I realize how important and vital it is to just simply wear a seatbelt.

These are the major symptoms to look out for when being concerned about traumatic brain injury. These are a list of symptoms to be aware of, and if you exhibit any or all of this *call the doctor or go to an emergency room!*

In adults:

1. Headaches or neck pain that is persistent and does not go away

2. Trouble concentrating or making decisions

3. Slow thinking, speaking, or reading

4. Getting lost or easily confused, and not being able to follow simple directions

5. Trouble remembering names

6. Feeling tired all of the time

7. Having little or no energy or drive

8. Mood swings

9. Changes in sleep patterns—trouble sleeping or sleeping too much

10. Lightheaded or dizzy or losing your balance

11. An urge to throw up

12. Increase in your sensitivity to lights, sounds, or distractions

13. Blurred vision or eyes that tired too easily

14. Ringing in the ears

15. Loss of sense of smell

Children

1. Tired or listless

2. Irritable or cranky or cannot be consoled

3. Changes in eating—will not eat or nurse

4. Changes in sleep patterns

5. Changes in the way the child plays

6. Changes in school performance

7. Loss of interest in favorite games or toys

8. Loss of interest in learning new skills

9. Loss of balance and unsteady walking

10. Vomiting

Causes of traumatic brain injury

There are many causes that contribute to traumatic brain Injury.

Traumatic brain injury is serious. You need to protect your brain, because without it you will not be able to function, think, or process information. You have only one brain, and you need to take precautions:

These are the primary causes of TBI:

1. Car accidents

2. Falls

3. Bicycle or motorcycle accidents

4. Sports participation

6. Assault/ gunshot wound

7. Violence

Your brain helps you understand and interpret information and the world around you. When your brain is injured there is a disruption in its ability to store, process, and retrieve information. It can also interfere with your ability to control your emotions and interact with others.

How do you know?

Many times we avoid the fact that we have a problem and tend to ignore it. DON'T! As with my head injury, I could not remember the incident—even now. I had trouble remembering the names of the people in the car and the names of my family members when they came to the hospital. Several days later, I found a shopping list in my bag that I'd written before we left. For some reason, reading that made things start to fall into place. It is common to forget what happened before an injury occurred, but symptoms cannot and should not be ignored.

How do I know if I need medical help?

Your injuries can range from the scalp and face, including lacerations, bruising, or abrasions. More common symptoms are:

1. Loss of consciousness

2. Concussion

3. Brain contusion

4. Skull fracture

5. Hematoma

However, there are numerous symptoms that you need to be aware of and address if they are also present:

- Headaches
- Lethargy
- Balance issues
- Nausea
- Fatigue
- Bad taste in the mouth
- Slurred speech

- Neck pain
- Anxiety
- Irritability
- Depression
- Difficulty concentrating
- Memory loss
- Trouble collecting thoughts
- Trouble sleeping
- Dilated pupils
- Drainage of blood or clear fluid from the nose or ears
- Weakness or numbness in the limbs

Other causes of traumatic brain injury

- Trucking accidents
- Defective products
- Unlawful alcohol sales
- Slipping and falling
- Work place injuries

Traumatic brain injuries and Alzheimer's

A head trauma and its role in the development of Alzheimer's are undergoing study. Most likely a serious head injury speeds up the onset of Alzheimer's disease. There may be a link between TBI and the onset of Alzheimer's years later. The main point is to address these injuries and follow the safety precautions to avoid them.

Final points:

Seniors and kids are prone to having the most accidents. 1.8 million seniors sixty-five and over are treated in the ER for falls.

Seniors: How can they prevent falls:

1. Exercise regularly

2. Install grab bars and non-slip mats

3. Hand rails should be installed

4. Make sure you have ample lighting

5. Be aware and careful of lose cords and extension cords. Be careful when you vacuum that you do not trip on the cord, and that cords are plugged in properly.

6. Be mindful of all medications with side effects, especially if you are going to drive or operate machinery.

7. Wear non-slip shoes and slippers

8. Make sure you get your vision tested

Preventing children from falling:

1. Do not leave a child alone or unattended in a tub/shower

2. Wall mounted non-accordion safety gates should be installed

3. Install doorknob covers, locks, stops, and door holders

4. Window guards should be installed

5. Never leave a side rail on a crib down—make sure it is secured and locked in place

6. Bunk beds should have guard rails placed on top bunks

7. In cars, use car seats

8. Supermarkets; Secure child in shopping cart with seatbelt

9. Make sure in restaurants you use a highchair that the child cannot slip out from the bottom, and there is something to secure them in the seat

10. Dry floors

11. Keep stairs clean

Remember these injuries can be avoided using the proper precautions. Traumatic brain injury is serious, and can leave lasting effects on adults, children, and seniors. Take precautions.

Characteristics of brain injury

How does it impair your senses or your thinking skills?

1. Slows down your thinking

2. Makes it difficult to complete tasks and jobs

3. Hard to remember things; memory and learning are hard

4. Trouble concentrating

5. Difficulty sequencing

6. You might disregard safety rules

7. Changes in your senses

8. You might have experienced these behavioral changes:

   - Anxiety
   - Impatience
   - Low self-esteem
   - Mood swings/changes
   - Difficulty coping
   - Self-centered
   - Headaches
   - Constant pain
   - Your balance might be off/walking
   - Appetite changes
   - Trouble swallowing
   - Seizures
   - Speech might be slurred
   - No speech
   - Bladder or bowel problems

Seek medical help if you notice marked changes. Hopefully symptoms will improve but they should not be ignored.

Frequently Asked Questions:
Traumatic Brain Injury

How does the Kessler Foundation work with patients with Brain Traumatic Injury?

Kids, adults, infants

1. What type of equipment is used to restore motor skills?

2. What exercises or therapy is used to restore brain function-reading, writing-math and language skills?

3. What type of physical therapy is done to restore movement?

4. What about occupational therapy?

5. What is done to restore mental brain function?

6. What type of traumatic brain injury is most prevalent?

7. What does the foundation do to work with these injuries, and which methods are most successful?

8. What, besides home accidents, sports injuries, or accidents in cars or moving vehicle, are the prime causes of TBI in teens and small children?

9. What medical reasons or causes might attribute to TBI?

If a person has a stroke or massive heart attack and falls on a hard floor, hitting their heads square on their face, would that result in TBI? What kind and how severe?

When someone loses oxygen to the brain for more than twenty-seven minutes and their lower brain function is still there:

1. In a small child could the higher function be restored?

2. In infants?

3. In adults?

When is it too late? What If someone tries to administer CPR and has no idea how chest compressions are done, and the person falls over on their face. Should they move the person or wait for 911?

What is hypoxia, and is it fatal?

How does a piece of plague break off in the heart, causing lack of oxygen to the brain?

Could a severe argument plus high blood pressure and heart palpitations cause a person to fall over and lose consciousness?

What would cause a person in good health to keel over?

Resources

www.allabouttbi.com

www.cdc.gov/TraumaticBraininjury

www.cdc.gov/HomeandRecreationalsafety/Playground-Injuries/playgroundinjuries-factsheet.htm#pl

http://www.michigan.gov/documents/mdch/Resources_for_
Persons_with_Brain_Injury_and_Their_Families_201404_7.
pdf

http://www.cdc.gov/injuryresponse/index.html

http://www.braininjury.com/symptoms.html

https://www.drbredesen.com/

PART THREE

Protecting the Elderly

Eldercare Abuse

What You Need To Know,
Understand and Learn to Prevent It

E ldercare abuse is prevalent in nursing homes, hospitals, and even at home. All too often aides, nurses and even caregivers are cruel to those who are frail, and unable to speak for themselves and fight back. Newspapers, online sites, and news commentators report these incidents on a daily basis, yet the abuse continues. Imagine that the abuser is someone you know—a family member you think you can trust, a spouse who is supposed to protect you, or health care worker.

How widespread or large is this problem?

If cases are not reported victims are not identified, so it is hard to state or answer this question. However, after visiting nursing homes, listening to some health care providers, and touring some hospitals, it was not hard to see. In one nursing home I witnessed the head administrator pushing a patient away from her when she tried to give her a hug. In two other homes many of the patients were lined up in wheelchairs in the hallway, either asleep, looking drugged, or just staring into outer space with no one talking or interacting with them.

Elder care abuse defined

This is no doubt that it is purposeful, intentional, and cruel, defined as the intentional or neglectful acts by someone trusted by a person—caregiver, spouse, aide, nurse—leading to harm of any elderly person who is vulnerable. Physical abuse or neglect can be emotional, psychological, verbal, and even financial. Exploitation, sexual abuse, and abandonment are forms of neglect and abuse. In some states self-neglect is considered abuse. Dealing with home care agencies for my mom has been a real eye-opener and totally enlightening. Replacement aides are often negligent, unfeeling, and in several cases abusive, both verbally and physically.

One specific incident comes to mind when the regular night aide was ill and the replacement came in. The day aides explained and remained for over one hour. My mom's condition and behaviors warranted twenty-four hour care and she could not eat, move, or speak for herself. The aide explained everything to this young arrogant person before leaving. About one hour later she called and claimed my mom had thrown her walker at her. That was a real laugh. My mom was sitting in her chair and watching television with a black and blue arm and wrist that she did not have before. My mom was fragile and could not lift a pencil by herself. The aide was sitting behind the table writing down what she claimed happened, and had a smirk on her face, letting me know she was not telling it straight. At that point I called the agency and demanded they send another aide, and that I was going to file a major complaint against her.

Elder care abuse shows itself in many forms:

- Physical
- Self-neglect
- Emotional
- Sexual
- Financial abuse
- Abandonment

How do you prevent elder abuse?

1. Report suspected mistreatment to local adult and protective agencies or police.

2. Keep in contact with neighbors and friends. Do not isolate the person. Be aware of what the caregiver/aides are doing.

3. Be aware of the possibility of abuse. Take note of elderly neighbors, especially if you see a change of attitude, or if they become withdrawn, nervous, fearful, or sad, and report it.

4. Contact your local area agency or aging office.

5. Volunteer to help in senior centers.

6. Learn about Elder Abuse World Day.

Resources

www.ncea.ava.gov

www.ncea-info@aoa.hhs.gov

www.ncea.aoa.gov

Nursing Home Abuse

Very prominent in the news is nursing home abuse. After visiting many homes to assess them or to visit friends of my mom and my aunt, who was in a hospice environment, and to see just what kind of care people received, I made my own decision as my mom's POA to keep her safe at home. That does not mean that I do not have to monitor her home care. It just means I am right there in case anything happens. Of course that puts the burden on me to monitor the aides, agency, and homecare services.

After visiting more than fifteen homes and seeing some of her friends in these facilities, I realized that I made the right decision. That is not to say that all nursing homes are neglectful or poorly run. It just means unless you are there on a daily basis, the person might not receive the care they need. Visibility is the key! When placing a parent or loved on in these facilities you need to do your homework first. Check out their website and learn about their services. Check out any complaints filed against the home. Visit at varied times—unannounced. Ask to see the patients that are the most seriously ill and need the most care. Observe how the staff interacts with these patients, and listen to the tone of their voices and observe their body language.

As you walk around observe the cleanliness of the place and the people to see if they are well groomed and cared for. See how they are dressed, or if too many are left to fend for themselves in their rooms because they cannot speak up or feed themselves. Observe what happens when a patient does not eat. Do they feed them or are they ignored?

Every home should have a daily plan or calendar posted with the day's activities. They should have copies to give visitors and family members too. What happens when a patient needs medical care not provided by the staff of the home? How fast do they call 911 for assistance? How fast do they call the family member? How are meds administered? Do they continue with the ones the patient is taking before entering the home, or do they change them, and if so why? Do they keep in contact with the patient's primary doctor, or is that doctor no longer kept informed? With my aunt my cousins take her to her own doctors, keeping her medications and physical needs the same.

Nursing home regulations require they participate in Medicare and Medicaid programs to conform to certain requirements for quality of care. Federal laws regulate quality of care, and New York State exacts care and the laws too. So why are there so many incidents of abuse? Nursing homes must conduct an initial comprehensive evaluation of each patient, and reassess periodically to see if there are any significant changes in the condition of the person. As with the home health aides and caregivers, even if they are family members, nursing homes are suppose to generate an individual plan of care specific for each patient, which must be documented in the person's file or clinical record. There are many homes that do not provide the required care, and patients deteriorate and die, violating federal and state laws. But then it is too late. It is even possible that the home submitted false claims to the government if they receive Medicare and Medicaid.

Suspect abuse?

Call Immediately — DON'T WAIT TO TAKE ACTION

- Pierro Law at 1-866-951-Plan
- Eldercare Locater at 1-800-677-1116
- 911

To report suspected abuse in a nursing home or long-term care facility, contact your state specific agency. To find the listing visit the Long-Term Care Ombudsman website at:

- http://www.ltcombudsman.org/ombudsman

- Contact the National Center on Elder Care Abuse/ NCEA c/o University of Delaware Center for Community Research and Service 297 Graham Hall, Newark, DE 19716

- www.cec.gov/ViolencePrevention/DELTA/index.html

Frequently Asked Questions: Elder Care Abuse

1. What is elder care abuse?
2. What are the warning signs?
3. What is self-neglect and what are the signs?
4. What makes an older adult vulnerable to abuse?
5. Who are these abusers? How can they be identified?
6. Are there criminal penalties for the abusers?
7. How many people are suffering from elder care abuse?
8. How can we make people more aware and how can I work to stop it?

True Stories

My Experiences with Caregiving

By Barbara Ehrentreu

My experience with care giving came when my husband had a heart attack that would require bypass surgery. He was transported to Westchester Medical Center by ambulance the day after the heart attack, since the hospital where he was first taken didn't do that kind of surgery.

Westchester Medical Center specialized in heart surgery, so I was very happy to see he was there. However, since he was also a patient at the Veteran's Administration, the resident doctor decided to have him transferred to a veteran's hospital facility. Unfortunately, that hospital didn't do bypass surgery.

When I found out about this, I was angry so I went to the ombudsman of the hospital and told them about this treatment. My husband was in an emergency and needed a bypass.

As soon as I saw the ombudsman and returned to my husband's room, I found he was getting an X-ray and being given materials for surgery. They did the surgery the following morning. If he had waited any longer, he would have died. His heart was beating at eleven percent, and his blood had turned black.

After the surgery he couldn't get off the breathing tube or wake up enough to be conscious, so they left the tube in him for almost two weeks. This caused him to contract bacterial pneumonia. The bacterial pneumonia required the hospital to isolate him, and we had to wear gowns and gloves when visiting him.

He was not really awake and rarely communicated with us. He knew my daughters and me, but since we couldn't speak with him we had no idea what he was thinking. When he was allowed to start to talk through the tracheotomy, he would grab my arm when I was leaving and say I should come early so we could talk. He did this several times, and I didn't know what he was talking about.

Later, when I needed to get his signature on a proxy form so I could pay our bills, the head of the nurses would not sign off on the paper. She said that she didn't think my husband was in his right mind. I was shocked, since he was such a logical and grounded person. So they had psychiatrists come in and interview him.

Was I surprised at his answers to their questions! He was asked to tell them what year it was, and he said 1964. Then they asked him where he was, and he said he was in a Vietnamese prisoner of war camp. The diagnosis was that he had a form of delirium.

Then he started to try to get out of bed all the time, and the hospital had to give him a one-on-one attendant. He would scream at them if they didn't do what he wanted. One time he got so angry with a male attendant who wouldn't give him his clothes that he kicked him. I couldn't believe that my husband did that.

I had to intervene several times during his treatment, because the VA wanted to transfer him and he wasn't ready to leave. He was given physical therapy to get him to walking better while in the hospital. Eventually, he came back to reality and returned to the logical person he had been.

Another time I had to be a caregiver was when my husband had very high calcium due to a sarcoidosis of his kidney. He was put in the hospital and given IV liquids to flush out the calcium. Then, when his level was almost normal, the doctors allowed him to go home and finish as an outpatient.

However, the doctors prescribed both high levels of Prednisone and a new kind of insulin, along with Ambien. In a few days, my husband was hallucinating, and then after an incident he was taken to the hospital again. There he continued to hallucinate and turned angry at night, screaming at the top of his lungs and getting out of bed, though he was very unsteady.

The nurses needed to restrain him, but he couldn't be contained. He was put on a bed alarm, but even then it didn't help. He would rave and so he was given a drug.

One night I went over to the hospital to see his behavior. While I was in his room, he got out of bed. When I wouldn't get his clothes for him, he slapped me. This brought the entire trauma staff to his room, and he was given a large does of medicine.

Barbara Ehrentreu is the author of *If I Could Be Like Jennifer Taylor,* MuseItUp Publishing. Visit her blog, Barbara's Meanderings at http://barbaraehrentreu.blogspot.com/

I Can't Breathe!

By Rev. Faith McDonald

In December of 1993, my husband, David, was electrocuted and I became his caregiver as a result. As a caregiver I would like to make a suggestion to all other caregivers, if I may—BREATHE!

I came to realize that David was not the only one whose life had been totally changed as a result of the electrocution, but our family as a whole was forced to go through life-altering changes. You just go into performance mode, much as soldiers do in a war—and believe me, you are in a war...just a silent, unknown one; not seen by many, invisible, painful, and scary. You lose yourself. But, in doing so, you find yourself.

I didn't know until my husband's accident that I had it within me to be a paramedic, an administrator, a nurse, a paralegal, a fundraiser, a P.R. person, a T.V. personality, and a hero, or at least that is what our local paper referred to me as. But those were the roles in which I found myself playing and operating. In my heart, in my mind, I was a wife, a mother, and a woman who was fearful, inadequate, and traumatized. It is amazing what a woman/man can be, when she or he is forced to be it in any given situation.

My advice would be to take a minute (if that is all that is afforded you) light a candle, sit in a quite place, without guilt, and BREATHE. Find people with whom you can talk who understand; talk therapy is essential. You can't give what you don't have.

My husband's condition has much improved. He has out-done everything that the doctors said he would never do. Caregiving is not a death sentence, but a rebirth into all of your and your loved one's possibilities.

Now What?

By Rev. Faith McDonald

The question that I am often asked at present time is, "Now what?"

The incident that occurred that thrust me into a caregiver's role happened when I was thirty-three years of age. I was a newlywed—we'd been married just a little over a year. (We've now been married for twenty-five years.)

My husband, David, was thirty-three years of age also when the accident occurred. Our birthdays are seventeen days apart. He was, and is, the love of my life.

As a result of a horrific above mentioned accident, he (David) became permanently disabled. He was electrocuted with 12,000 volts of electricity for 10 and 1/2 seconds, which changed our lives forever. Yes, life can change forever that quickly, in a blink of an eye.

During David's hospital stay at a burn unit that was then in Chattanooga TN., I was being forced to make life changing, life altering decisions for a man I barely knew, in regards to the time we knew each other chronologically, However, I did know him, on a very deep level, spiritually

I was making decisions for him that his family neither agreed with nor understood—because he and I are people of faith and they (his family) were and are very carnal. That stress alone and the battles that we fought were and are mind-boggling.

I am now 58 years of age. It is 25 years later and I now feel the impact of this journey and how it has affected me—the stress, weight gain, PTSD, CFS, FM, complicated migraine headaches, and acute anxiety.

No one told me the cost. There was no manual or, if there was, I didn't know about it. No one shared with me the wealth of information that this book, the one that you are now reading, conveys. Sharing this wellspring of information with you, we do, "Because We Care."

Our home became a place of self-employment. I had to do "at home" jobs in order to care for my husband.

Stress takes it toll on marriages, on families, and individuals, both the patient and the caregiver.

In the beginning, right after David's accident, many rallied around us to help. Months into it, help was often offered but less frequently, and then eventually not at all. Most people didn't understand that this was a life sentence for us.

My husband is still disabled but has a strong spirit, and as many are forced to do, learned to adapt to his new way of life as much as one can. Now I'm the one on disability, learning new ways to cope and to adapt.

The fires that we go through in life, shape us.

I'm learning self-care, self-love, and yes, even what some might call selfishness, for lack of a better word.

Better years are ahead of me. I am still a very caring person. For the first time in my life, I care about ME!

I'm learning to give the same love, attention, and affection that I have given all my life to so many others to myself. As a child, I was a caregiver for my sick father, for my hurting mother, and for many years, offered full time ministry to hundreds upon hundreds of others.

Now what? The above is what I am asking of you. Take care of yourself. I know many won't understand it. Learn to say no without explaining yourself or feeling guilty. People will use you until they use you up. Set boundaries. Love yourself.

My husband and I are very much in love, and he "cares for me" deeply. The rolls have reversed.

My husband, David, although he fights his own challenges, and has overcome much adversity, is a daily inspiration to me. We have taken this journey both together and separately. We are grateful for one another, and pray we grow old together gracefully.

Take good care of yourself and each other.

True story about elder care abuse

By Dellani Oakes

My mother is a very independent woman, who has been forced by circumstances and failing memory to be completely dependent. It was not an easy transition, and is still difficult for her. For quite some time, she lived on her own, but finally decided to move to a retirement community in Ohio. Both her sisters lived there, so it seemed the ideal choice. It was, until one sister died and the other moved closer to her daughter. My mother, still in her own apartment, was far from my sister and me.

I live in Florida, and had hoped to get Mom to move down here, but she put her foot down. "I hate Florida!" Since she was still able to cope on her own, we didn't push. She didn't want to move near my sister in Kansas, either, so again, we didn't push.

There came the time, shortly after her ninetieth birthday, when she fell and broke her hip a second time. The repair work was botched, and she was in a great deal of pain afterward.

Therapists concluded that she would probably never be able to walk again. Another surgeon was consulted, but he refused to do the surgery to repair what the other doctor messed up. After a long discussion between Mom, my sister, and me, we determined he was right. The surgery would be extensive, nearly nine hours, if all went well. For a woman her age to be under anesthetic that long was very risky. She resigned herself to being in the chair. Though she was still able to stand, she couldn't for long, and she grew much weaker.

My sister and I weren't close enough to check up on her. She had no family nearby, though our cousins and children visited when they could. We weren't in the position to fly or drive up to see her more than once a year, each. This put her in the prime position for neglect by the nursing home, as did her creeping dementia.

We noticed little things over the phone; forgetting what she was talking about, the inability to pull the right words together, confusing us or our children. Since she was ninety-three, we could understand the decline. Unfortunately, we had no idea how far she had fallen until I visited her in October of 2013.

Normally I went up for her birthday in mid-September, but my husband's parents, who were both failing, needed him. When he got back from his visit with them, I flew to Ohio. Mom was in good spirits, but I could tell she was having difficulty. After a long chat with the women who cleaned her room, and a couple of others who worked there, I started to get a much clearer picture. They were worried that she wasn't eating as she should, and she was in grave danger of another fall. Yes, she had a panic button, but she wouldn't wear it at night. Instead, she hung it nearly five feet from her bed. No clear reason for that, it's just what she did. Though I tried to move it closer, she would put it back in the original place.

After a chat with the nursing staff, which didn't get me much of anywhere, I finally got a list of her medications and did some exploring. The Internet is an amazing tool. I was concerned that some of her issues were brought on by medication interactions or side effects. The two biggest culprits were Ativan and Vicodin.

I've never taken Ativan, which is used predominantly to treat anxiety. It's also a nursing home's drug of choice to keep a patient subdued. I have taken Vicodin, and it does nasty things to me. Yes, it's a moderately effective pain relief medication, but I don't like how it makes me feel. Judging by the fact it also makes my daughter uncomfortable, I thought "Hey, maybe it's genetic!"

I did some searching on the official Vicodin and Ativan sites. Under contraindications and drug interactions, it said, to paraphrase, that these two medications should NEVER be taken together. Not that it was okay, once in awhile. Not that it was just fine and dandy. NEVER. I approached the nursing staff with my concerns. I ran off the lists of ill effects from both drugs, and highlighted the ones my mother exhibited. Most of them.

They nodded and looked wide-eyed, and no one did anything. One nurse did say, "Well, she's been fine so far."

"You think that's okay?" I asked, borderline furious. "Because she's been fine so far, that's all right? What about when she's not fine, and it kills her? You can say on the death certificate, 'Well, she was fine yesterday!'"

She blinked a lot and did nothing. Finally, I bugged them so much they gave us an appointment with the in-house P.A.

Let me preface this next anecdote with this: My mother never insults people. She might be critical, but she's not offensive. She addresses people by their names, and doesn't refer to anyone with insulting epithets. EVER. She called the P.A. "The stupid fat girl." She couldn't remember her name, but boy did she know who that young woman was! Already prepared for trouble, I took her to her appointment.

We went through the basic exam, with the P.A. speaking to Mom like a child. What makes people thing that the elderly want to be spoken to as if they are mentally deficient three year olds? My mother is a brilliant woman, much smarter, even in her diminished capacity, than *the stupid fat girl*. She had that patient tone, as if Mom were going to get riled and start throwing things. Truth be told, I was ready to throw things when we were done.

I got nothing from her. I wanted her off the Ativan. I conceded that she needed the Vicodin, though I thought they needed to find something else to put her on. She finally decided to put her on Ibuprofen, but didn't want to take her off the Ativan until she checked with the doctor.

She didn't check with the doctor. She stalled and stuttered, so I called his office, and was put off by the staff. I never was able to speak to the man. I never was able to get her off the Ativan. Absolutely no one would listen to me, though my sister and I both hold medical power of attorney.

As if this weren't bad enough, they had gotten in a new medication, which was supposed to help her dementia. The Exelon Patch (rivastigmine transdermal system), is supposed to be good for people with dementia from Alzheimer's or Parkinson's, neither of which my mother had been diagnosed with. It's very expensive, and *the stupid fat girl* was really excited that it had finally been cleared by the insurance company.

Mother agreed to let them try it, and they put it on her about 3:00 in the afternoon. By dinnertime, I barely recognized my mother. The sparkle that made her shine was a dull sheen. I took her to the cafeteria for dinner, and we went to order at the window.

"What do you want to eat, Mom?" This was always a big decision, and we had fun discussing what we wanted. I read off the specials on the board outside.

"I don't care."

My mother always cares what she eats. She's not picky, but she likes that modicum of control over her meal.

"Do you want soup and salad?"

"I don't care."

"You want to try the meat loaf? It looks good."

"I don't care."

I placed our order and took her to a nearby table to wait for me. Already, the workers noticed her lack of animation. My mother always stopped to chat with everyone. They all knew her by name, and she always recognized voices, (her vision is very poor) even if she didn't know names. The woman at the cash register gave me a wide-eyed stare when I went up to pay.

"Is she okay?" she whispered. "She didn't even know me when I went to say hello. She always knows me. She even remembers my name, and asks after my kids."

I told her what they'd put on her, and her expression became deeply worried. "Oh."

She didn't say anything else, but I could see she was concerned. Mom's friends stopped at the table to say hello, but she didn't respond. She asked me several times what she was eating, and finally stopped. I ended up feeding my mother. I don't think she even noticed.

Since she was exhausted by that time, we went to her apartment, and I stayed while she got ready for bed. The process took her extra long, because she kept forgetting what she was doing. I made sure she went to the toilet and brushed her teeth. I washed her face for her, and helped her change into her gown. She got into bed with her chair nearby, and I left.

I spent an uneasy night, and went to check on her very early the next day. I found her wrapped in her afghan, soaking wet with urine, nearly freezing. The room was very cold, because the temperature had dropped during the night. I got her cleaned up as best I could and rushed her down to the clinic.

"Take it off her!" I told the nurse as soon as I walked in the door. "Take it off and don't put it on her ever again!"

To say they were shocked was an understatement. None of them wanted to help me, so I told them to give me gloves so I could do it myself. One of the nurses, who was kind of a bitch, came over. She was probably my least favorite of the nursing staff, but she was willing to do it. She peeled the patch off my mother's shoulder and saw how red and raw the skin was beneath it. Her eyes clouded when she saw that. Ever so gently, she washed it with Betadine and dried it with gauze, before rubbing some Benadryl cream over it.

"I'm so sorry," she whispered. I thought she was going to cry. She spoke very gently to my mother, asking how she was.

Mom didn't respond. She looked at her, and didn't even smile. The nurses all got very busy.

"We don't want this any more," I told her again. "I want you to add it to her file, she refuses this medication."

"She needs to do that herself," another of the nurses said.

"I'm refusing for her. You check your paperwork, you'll see that I can."

She started to get her back up, so I turned to my mother. "Mom, do you want that medication anymore?"

"No!" It was the clearest she'd spoken since the prior afternoon.

I took her to breakfast and got her a large cup of coffee. We didn't leave the cafeteria until she'd had two cups. I had to feed her the first part of the meal, but she started to perk up a little bit by the time we were done. When we went back to the clinic for her evening medication, she stated very clearly that they could throw the rest of the medication away.

"Some medications take some getting used to," one foolish woman said.

"I refuse to get used to that," Mom replied. "No more."

I made sure they entered it into her record. They weren't too happy with me standing there, looking over their shoulders, while they did it. It took almost twenty-four hours for her to spring back from that medication.

I was there ten days, and felt the entire time as if I were knocking my head against a brick wall. I had one small victory with the Vicodin, but it felt like nothing. I was glad I was there for the Exelon Patch fiasco. I can't even imagine what would have happened if I hadn't been.

As it turned out, my victory over the Vicodin was short lived. The day after I left, they gave it to my mother again. All the fighting with the nurses, talking to the P.A., and my conversations with the social worker did no good. Shortly after this mess, we moved our mother to a facility only twenty minutes from my sister. No one is trying to drug her into submission, and they caught the Vicodin and Ativan conflict as soon as her paperwork was transferred.

Our mother suffered greatly at the hands of uncaring medical staff, but now she is well cared for. She will be 99 in September. Though she is still in a wheelchair and has diminished mental capacity, she isn't being mistreated. That, of itself, is the greatest gift.

Find Dellani Oakes at Blog Talk Radio, Dellani's Tea Time, and her blog at http://writersanctuary.blogspot.com/

Closing Remarks

Think about how many people need help and do not have family members to speak for them or take care of them. Think about how you can make a positive difference in someone's life: Volunteer: Become A Caregiver. Learn how to protect yourself, your family and your children from Traumatic Brain Injury. Protecting the Elderly is so vital and important. Learn the Causes and Signs of Eldercare Abuse and help STOP IT!

Use this book as your guide.

This book is dedicated to two of the most amazing women in my life: My sister, Marcia Wallach who died from traumatic brain injury on July 8, 2010 and my mom, who made me strong, kind, responsible and caring: Ruth Swerdloff who passed away on March 7, 2010. My mom had Alzheimer's and many other heart related illnesses. She was my voice growing up and I was hers for the past 10 years. If I had to do it again I would.

Special thank you to the nurses on 9 North and 8 North in Albert Einstein Hospital in the Bronx for taking care of my mom and showing such understanding and compassion to all of your patients. To Daria Smith the nurse case manager and Anne the manager on 8 North you are so special and thank you for understanding my mom's needs and helping me when I needed your assistance.

www.ingramcontent.com/pod-product-compliance
Lightning Source LLC
Chambersburg PA
CBHW071237020426
42333CB00015B/1516